BODY SCRUBS

30 Organic Homemade Body And Face Scrubs

The Best All-Natural Recipes For Soft, Radiant And Youthful Skin

Miranda Ross

TABLE OF CONTENTS

INTRODUCTION 5
THE ABCS OF SCRUBS 8
    WHY SCRUB IS NECESSARY TO HAVE RADIANT SKIN? 9
    DOES YOUR SKIN NEEDS TO BE SCRUBBED? 9
EXFOLIATION CURES SKIN DISEASES 11
BENEFITS OF HOMEMADE SCRUBS 17
HOMEMADE SCRUB RECIPES 19
    STRAWBERRY & COCONUT OIL 20
    ALMOND & HONEY 22
    GRAM FLOUR & YOGURT 24
    ORANGE & KIWI 26
    STRAWBERRY & BROWN SUGAR 28
    WHEAT BRAN & FLAX-SEED 29
    CINNAMON & BROWN SUGAR 31
    CUCUMBER & ORANGE 32
    ALOE VERA & HONEY 34
    APRICOT & WALNUT 36
    LEMON & ALMOND 38
    TOMATO & SEA SALT 40
    VANILLA, COFFEE & SUGAR 42
    LEMONGRASS & OLIVE OIL 44
    BANANA, OATS & HONEY 46

Banana & Brown Sugar	48
Pomegranate & Sugar	50
Watermelon & Mint	51
Banana & Yogurt	53
Blueberry & Green Tea	55
Sugar, Lemon & Olive Oil	56
Orange & Oatmeal	57
Egg Shell & Cream	59
Sea Salt & Olive Oil	60
Coffee & Honey	61
Coconut & Brown Sugar	62
Oats, Honey & Grapefruit	63
Lemon, Sugar & Honey	65
Kiwi & Sugar	66
Strawberry, Honey & Almond	67
CONCLUSION	**69**

INTRODUCTION

This book contains 30 effective homemade facial and body scrubs recipes. The recipes mentioned in this book are simple and easy to be made with no side effects. Moreover, all the homemade scrubs recipes contains natural ingredients, which in all forms and contexts are good for human skin.

Furthermore, this book contains general information regarding why scrubs are important to have fresh, lively and glowing skin. Benefits of scrubs are also being included so that this book could help people in knowing every basic thing about facial and body scrubs.

I hope you enjoy it!

© **Copyright 2015 by Miranda Ross - All rights reserved.**

This document is geared towards providing exact and reliable information in regards to the topic and issue covered. The publication is sold with the idea that the publisher is not required to render accounting, officially permitted, or otherwise, qualified services. If advice is necessary, legal or professional, a practiced individual in the profession should be ordered.

From a Declaration of Principles which was accepted and approved equally by a Committee of the American Bar Association and a Committee of Publishers and Associations.

In no way is it legal to reproduce, duplicate, or transmit any part of this document in either electronic means or in printed format. Recording of this publication is strictly prohibited and any storage of this document is not allowed unless with written permission from the publisher. All rights reserved.

The information provided herein is stated to be truthful and consistent, in that any liability, in terms of inattention or otherwise, by any usage or abuse of any policies, processes, or directions contained within is the solitary and utter responsibility of the recipient reader. Under no circumstances will any legal responsibility or blame be held against the publisher for any reparation, damages, or monetary loss due to the information herein, either directly or indirectly.

Respective authors own all copyrights not held by the publisher.

The information herein is offered for informational purposes solely, and is universal as so. The presentation of the information is without contract or any type of guarantee assurance.

The trademarks that are used are without any consent, and the publication of the trademark is without permission or backing by the trademark owner. All trademarks and brands within this book are for clarifying purposes only and are the owned by the owners themselves, not affiliated with this document.

DISCLAIMER: The purpose of this book is to provide information only. The information, though believed to be entirely accurate, is NOT a substitution for medical, psychological or professional advice, diagnosis or treatment. The author recommends that you seek the advice of your physician or other qualified health care provider to present them with questions you may have regarding any medical condition. Advice from your trusted, professional medical advisor should always supersede information presented in this book.

THE ABCS OF SCRUBS

Human skin functions in such a way that it needs to be exfoliated every once in a while. As we grow in age, our skin grows up too. Some cells die and some other are born, thus, gives new surface to our skin. The dead cells remain on the skin until and unless they are removed. The dead cells are likely to form a layer on our skin if they are not removed, thus, making the new surface of our skin invisible. Moreover, as dead cells forms a complete layer over the new skin, the skin looks like dead and rough. So, to have a radiant skin, it is important that the dead cells are removed from the skin every once in a while.

Moreover, our skin gets exposed to the pollution everyday as we go outside. The pollution makes our skin dull and dead if it is not cleaned up from skin. So, it is important to have a moment to cleanse the skin whenever skin is exposed to pollution. If the skin is washed instantly, then it is less likely that the skin would eventually end up as rough and dead. But, if it isn't cleaned right away, then scrub becomes a must for cleansing of human skin.

WHY SCRUB IS NECESSARY TO HAVE RADIANT SKIN?

Scrubs consists of various natural oils and ingredients which gives life to human skin. Just like we need oxygen, our skin needs it too. When dead cells forms layers over our skin, fresh layer of skin doesn't get much oxygen, and eventually, it is affected negatively. Partial negative effects are due to the dead cells' layers and the remaining partial effects are due to the lack of oxygen that our skin collects. All these things combine and makes our skin rough and dull. So, in such situation, scrubs serves as lifesaving hope for our skin. They slowly and gradually removes dead cells in the first stage, then they clear up the pores and clears the skin so that it could have sufficient oxygen, and at last, scrubs give a refreshing look, a life and a glow to our skin.

DOES YOUR SKIN NEEDS TO BE SCRUBBED?

Natural functioning of human skin works the same way for all of us. This question can be accurately answered if we specify the duration of time in which human skins needs to be scrubbed. The duration of time period in which one must scrub his or her skin, varies from person to person, depending upon the skin type and current state. The more you have dull skin, the more frequently you need to scrub it up. You will eventually observe that your skin starts to glow after you scrub it a few times.

Your skin definitely needs to be scrubbed of course. Just try to figure out how often you have to scrub it. Even if you have perfect skin, you should scrub it at least once in a week.
Scrubbing your skin should be a priority for you if you want to keep your skin glowing and young. Moreover, scrubs will open up all the clogged pores of your skin and increase the blood circulation, hence, making it more beautiful and attractive.
So, you should scrub your skin regularly and stay beautiful and young!

EXFOLIATION CURES SKIN DISEASES

WHAT IS SKIN EXFOLIATION?

The removal of upper layer of dry, dead and damaged skin cells is called skin exfoliation.

SIGNIFICANCE OF EXFOLIATION

If you want your skin to be healthy, fresh, shiny and glowing all the time, then exfoliation is considered to be one of the best techniques. You can perform exfoliation on your skin to get rid of certain skin problems. Even the estheticians give positive statements about exfoliation and consider it the skin transformer.

WHAT KIND OF SKIN CARE PROBLEMS ARE ADDRESSED BY EXFOLIATION?

Exfoliation addresses many types of skin care problems. These problems include the following.

Blemished Skin

Exfoliation is the main center of a home care or remedial program. Acne products are suggested more often for the oily skin, which prove to be harsh for the skin. These products tend to dry out the skin completely. Although, they destroy the bacteria too, yet, most of the times, result in extreme irritability of the skin and future breakouts of the skin. Do you know why this happens? It happens because your skin gets over-dried and the cells of the dry skin starts accumulating on the surface layer. This layer becomes a barrier inside which, the oil is trapped in the skin. Thus, a cycle of new breakouts begins. If you don't want to have any mark of bacteria on your skin while exfoliating, you can use BHA Clarifying serum or likewise products. Such serums clean out clogged pores deeply and marvelously work to give you a fresh and newly refined clarity and smoothness.

Post-Breakout Red or Dark Marks

The blemishes do not cause the actual problem, rather the red or dark marks left on the skin after the healing of breakout are the source of real concern. If you increase your exfoliation, these post-breakout marks can be faded away. Enhance the removal of the surface dead cells and you will ultimately get rid of the dark marks. Thus, healthy new skin cells are formed, resulting in more even skin tone with reduced scarring. Post-Breakout Fading Gel is recommended to face away the left over scars.

Clogged Pores

Clogged pores, wrongly known as infected blemishes, are actually the little clogged bumps on the skin, blackheads or whiteheads. Same treatment, as for blemished skin is given in the case of clogged pores. Remove the surface dead layer of the skin cells, and this would cause less oil entrapment and congestion in the pores. Wash with cleansing gels to clear out clogged pores.

Hyperpigmentation

Hormonal changes, genetics, pregnancy and age are the main sources of hyperpigmentation, causing brown spots on the skin, which become darker and apparent with time. Pigmented cells are broken down by exfoliation and are eventually faded.

Dry Skin

Skin is vulnerable to be attacked by dryness in winters. In such cases, people start loading on heavier creams, increasing the dry skin cell buildup. So, increase your exfoliation to get rid of the dry skin and moisturize the new skin cells.

Uneven skin

If you want an even and smooth skin, then you need to exfoliate.

Wrinkles

Natural exfoliation process of the skin slows down as the skin ages. Exfoliants repair the lower layers, which is the house for collagen and elastin, and regular use leads to younger and smoother skin.

WHEN SHOULD YOU EXFOLIATE?

Two types of exfoliants are known, which are mentioned below.

Chemical exfoliants

Ingredients such as Glycolic acid, BHA and AHAs (Alpha Hydroxy Acids), and enzymes found in pumpkin, pineapple and papaya fall in the category of chemical exfoliants.

Physical exfoliants

Facial brushes, facial scrubs and sponges are listed in the category of physical exfoliants. Here, you have to do the needful yourself.

Chemical and physical exfoliants combined give the best results for your skin.

Use mild alcohol-free Glycolic Acid Serum or AHAs as night creams, taking three nights on and the other three off. You provide the best exfoliation for your skin this way, giving break to your skin as well. You can combine this with a mild facial scrub to vanish the dissolved skin cells. This combination can be used twice a week.

In order to select the best exfoliants for your skin, inspect and analyze your skin type carefully and make the best recommended exfoliating product for your skin on your own.

BENEFICIAL EXFOLIATING TREATMENTS

Many professional exfoliating treatments are advantageous for your skin, one of which includes bio brasion offered by many skin care spas. Bio brasion is actually a low-suction and crystal-free abrasion system that has customized levels of exfoliation using gentle vibration. Interchangeable and unique tips are passed across the surface of the skin slowly upwards, which then lift off the outermost damaged and dry skin, and the new healthy layers beneath are revealed. This, bio brasion is known as the next generation of microdermabrasion. Other professional treatments include chemical peels, ultrasonic exfoliation and enzyme peels. These methods provide your skin with more intense and deep exfoliation.

You should aim at exfoliating the skin to a maximum possible extent with minimum irritation. Give your skin a boost but not on daily basis.

TEST FOR EXFOLIATION REQUIREMENT

A simple test can be performed at home to check if you need exfoliation. Take a clear piece of tape and stick it on your forehead. Rub it and then, remove it from your forehead. If you see tiny pieces of flaky skin, that means you have dead and dry cells on your skin surface and therefore, your skin needs exfoliation in order to stay healthy, even and fresh.

All the treatments mentioned above have side effects on your skin. Some of them makes the skin allergic and irritable, while others may speed up the loosening of skin with aging. So, to avoid these side effects, we are sharing 30 homemade recipes of scrubs in the next chapters so that you can prepare your own scrub, 100% safe for your skin.

BENEFITS OF HOMEMADE SCRUBS

Homemade scrubs are best source of cleansing your skin from all the dirt and the dead cells just in a single go. Homemade scrubs are made completely out of natural ingredients so they don't have any side effects. They are not only efficient in removing dead cells, but also makes your skin glow as natural ingredients of homemade scrubs have various oils and vitamins that are a must for a beautiful skin. Following are some to the point benefits of homemade scrubs.

- Homemade scrubs make your skin smoother instantly. If you don't get time to get your skin scrubbed daily, you can just scrub it every once in a while when you feel your skin gets a bit dull. Scrub will bring an instant glow and freshness to your skin.
- Scrubs helps to reduce clogged pores and levels breakouts.

- Scrubs are helpful for improved collagen production in human skin.
- Scrubs even the tome of your skin complexion.
- Scrubs are helpful to reduce brown spots from human skin.
- Scrubs also helps to decrease and slowly eliminate acne scars left after breakout.
- Scrubs reduces dryness and flakiness to a very noticeable extent.
- As scrubs removes dead cells from skin, moisturizers and other serums have a great effect on skin because fresh layer of skin comes directly in contact with them.
- Scrubs take away pollution from your skin, even from the deeper pores of it, so it prevents pimples.

Scrubs are not only beneficial for human skin, but essential too. If you want to stay young and you want to look fresh and lively, you must scrub your skin every once in a while.

HOMEMADE SCRUB RECIPES

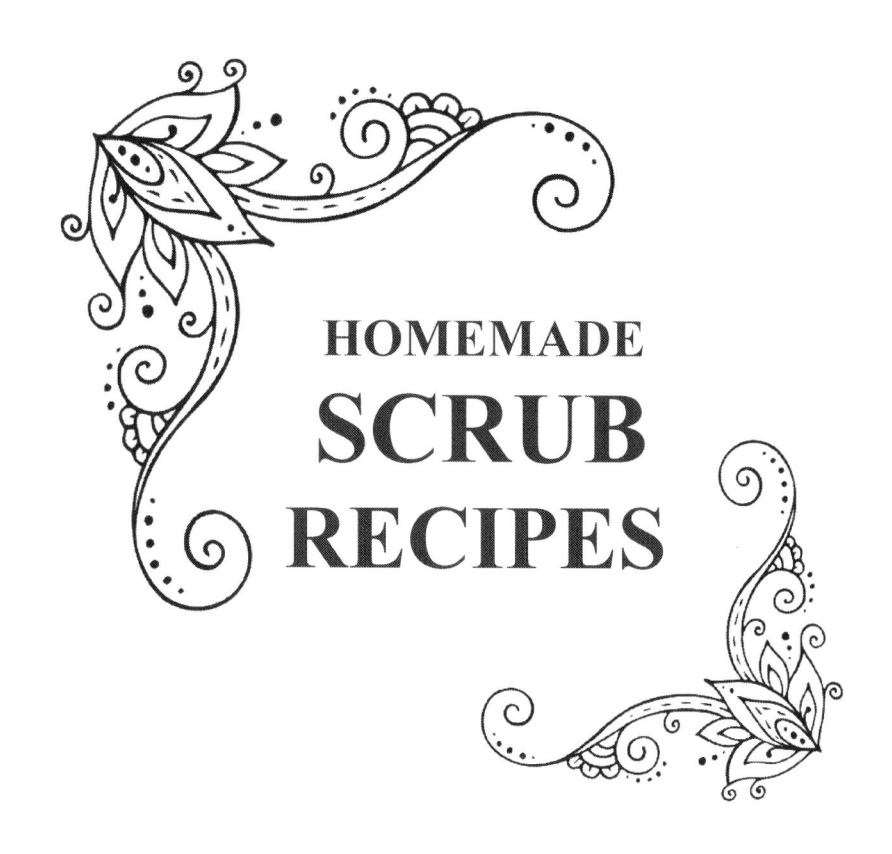

Here are 30 easy recipes that can be prepared within a few minutes and applied on skin for achieving best results. You can try them out in home as these are 100% safe for your skin.

Strawberry & Coconut Oil

Ingredients

- 2 - 3 strawberries
- 3 – 4 drops of coconut oil
- 1 teaspoon sugar

Method

1. Blend the strawberries just enough to let the seeds remain whole.
2. Add the coconut oil and sugar.
3. Mix all ingredients.

TO USE

- **ON YOUR FACE:** Apply to the face and massage in circular motions for 1 minute. Rinse well with water.
- **ON YOUR HANDS:** Massage into your hands and fingernails for 30 seconds. Rinse well.

*Use on the same day

Strawberries are best for skin because they contain vitamin C, antioxidants, exfoliants and salicylic acid.

Almond & Honey

Ingredients

- ½ teaspoon milk
- 5 grams of almonds
- 3 drops of lavender oil
- 1 teaspoon honey

Method

1. Grind the almonds to attain a powder form.
2. Mix the milk with the powered almonds.
3. Add the lavender oil and honey to the above mixture.
4. Mix well.

TO USE

- **ON YOUR FACE:** Apply to the face for 15 minutes. Let it dry before rubbing. Massage in circular motions for 30 seconds. Rinse well with warm water.
- **ON YOUR HANDS:** Massage into your hands and fingernails for 30 seconds. Rinse well with warm water.

*Use on the same day

Almonds are good for skin because they contain vitamin E and antioxidants.

Gram Flour & Yogurt

Ingredients

- 1 teaspoon gram flour
- ½ teaspoon fresh lemon juice
- 1 tablespoon yogurt

Method

1. Mix together gram flour and yogurt to form a thick paste.
2. Squeeze in the lemon juice from fresh lemon.
3. Mix well.

TO USE

- **ON YOUR FACE:** Apply to the face for 15 minutes. Let it dry before rubbing. Massage with wet hands in circular motions for 30 seconds. Rinse well with warm water and moisturize.
- **ON YOUR HANDS:** Massage into your hands and fingernails for 30 seconds. Rinse well with warm water.

*Use on the same day

Gram flour keeps skin lively, radiant and give it instant whitening.

Orange & Kiwi

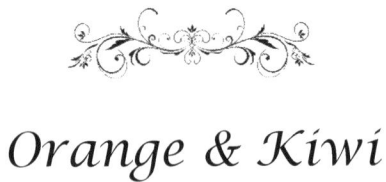

Ingredients

- 5 drops of fresh orange juice or orange essential oil
- 1 kiwi (the flesh of the kiwi)
- 1 tablespoon yogurt
- 3-4 drops of olive oil

Method

1. Mash the kiwi in a bowl that the seeds remain whole.
2. Squeeze in a few drops of orange juice or orange essential oil.
3. Add the yogurt.
4. Finally add a few drops of olive oil.
5. Mix all ingredients well.

TO USE

- ON YOUR FACE: Apply to the face and massage in circular motions for 30 seconds. Rinse well with water.

- ON YOUR HANDS: Massage into your hands and fingernails for 30 seconds. Rinse well.
- ON YOUR BODY: Massage in circular motions for a few minutes. Rinse well.

Remember, you can double or triple ingredients to make more scrub.

*Use on the same day

Orange peel has a great content of vitamin C, even greater than the fruit itself. So its scrub brings instant positive results over our skin. Kiwi has vitamin C, vitamin E and antioxidants which bring life to our skin and make it younger and smoother.

Strawberry & Brown Sugar

Ingredients

- 5 strawberries
- ½ teaspoon of fresh lemon juice
- 1-2 tablespoons brown sugar
- 2 tablespoons honey

Method

1. Mash strawberries in a food processor.
2. Add the honey and lemon juice. Mix well.
3. In the end, add brown sugar to make a thick paste.

TO USE

- ON YOUR FACE: Apply to the face and massage in circular motions for 1 minute. Rinse well with water.
- ON YOUR HANDS: Massage into your hands and fingernails for 1 minute. Rinse well with warm water.

*Use on the same day

Wheat Bran & Flax-Seed

Ingredients

- 4 teaspoons wheat bran
- 4 teaspoons flax-seed
- 1 teaspoon warm water
- 1 teaspoon honey

Method

1. Mix all ingredients together.

TO USE

- **ON YOUR FACE:** Apply to the face and let it dry for 15 minutes. Massage in circular motions (with wet hands) for 30 seconds. Rinse well with water.
- **ON YOUR HANDS:** Massage into your hands and fingernails for 1 minute. Rinse well with warm water.
- **ON YOUR LEGS AND FEET:** Massage in circular motions for 1 minute. Rinse well.

*Use on the same day

Flax-seed is beneficial for erasing signs of aging from human skin.

Cinnamon & Brown Sugar

Ingredients
- 1 cup of brown sugar
- ½ cup coconut oil
- ½ teaspoon cinnamon
- ½ teaspoon vitamin E oil

Method
1. Mix all ingredients.
2. Store in an air-tight container and keep it in fridge.

TO USE
- ON YOUR HANDS: Massage into your hands and fingernails for 1 minute. Rinse well with warm water.
- ON YOUR LEGS AND FEET: Massage in circular motions for 1 minute. Rinse well.
- ON YOUR BODY: Massage in circular motions for a few minutes. Rinse well.

*Scrub needs to be used within a month

Cucumber & Orange

Ingredients

- 1 small cucumber
- 1 teaspoon dried orange peel
- 4-5 drops of olive oil

Method

1. Squeeze out the cucumber pulp in a bowl and beat well.
2. Add the powdered orange peel.
3. Pour 4-5 drops of olive oil and mix well.

TO USE

- **ON YOUR FACE:** Apply to the face and massage in circular motions for 1 minute. Rinse well with water.
- **ON YOUR HANDS:** Massage into your hands and fingernails for 1 minute. Rinse well with warm water.

*Use on the same day

Cucumber is good for skin because it keeps the skin hydrated and ultimately keeps it young and glowing.

Aloe Vera & Honey

Ingredients

- 2 tablespoons Aloe Vera gel
- 1 teaspoon baking soda
- 2 tablespoons honey

Method

1. Squeeze out about 2 tablespoons of the Aloe Vera gel in a bowl.
2. Add the honey and baking soda.
3. Mix all ingredients.

TO USE

- ON YOUR FACE: Apply to the face and massage in circular motions for 1 minute. Rinse well with water.
- ON YOUR HANDS: Massage into your hands and fingernails for 1 minute. Rinse well.
- ON YOUR LEGS AND FEET: Massage in circular motions for a few minutes. Rinse well with warm water.

*Use on the same day

Honey is good for your skin because it acts as anti-aging. Moreover, it helps to protect your skin from absorbing extra UV rays hence making it less likely to be affected by diseases like cancer or allergies.

Apricot & Walnut

Ingredients

- 3-4 apricots
- 4 pieces of walnut shell
- 2 tablespoons honey
- 1 teaspoon apricot kernel oil or almond oil

Method

1. Peel off the outer skin of the fruit and then puree it in a blender. You can use a cheese grater and make a paste.
2. Grind walnut shell to form a powder and add to the apricot puree. You can use the amount of powder as per your convenience.
3. Add the honey.
4. Pour the oil just to retain the moisture of the skin.
5. Mix all ingredients well.

TO USE

- ON YOUR HANDS: Massage into your hands and fingernails for 1 minute. Rinse well with warm water.
- ON YOUR LEGS AND FEET: Massage in circular motions for a few minutes. Rinse well.
- ON YOUR BODY: Massage in circular motions for a few minutes. Rinse well.

Optional: Instead of walnut shell you can make the apricot kernel powder. Roast the seeds in the sunlight for 2 – 3 days. Once the seeds become dry, break the outer shell using a nutshell breaker and get kernels. Use a grinder to grind the kernels to a fine powder.

*Use on the same day

Apricot is rich in vitamin C and vitamin E so it keeps skin young, fresh and lively.

Lemon & Almond

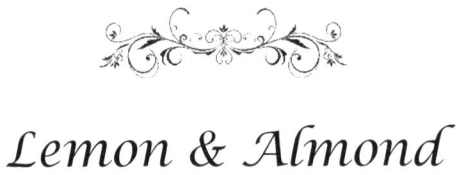

Ingredients
- 1/2 cup brown sugar
- ½ cup almond oil
- 6 drops of lemon essential oil
- ½ teaspoon vitamin E oil

Method
1. Mix all the ingredients.
2. Store in an air-tight container and keep it in fridge.

TO USE
- ON YOUR FACE: Apply to the face and massage in circular motions for 1 minute. Rinse well with water.
- ON YOUR HANDS: Massage into your hands and fingernails for 1 minute. Rinse well with warm water.
- ON YOUR LEGS AND FEET: Massage in circular motions for a few minutes. Rinse well.
- ON YOUR BODY: Massage in circular motions for a few minutes. Rinse well and moisturize.

*Scrub needs to be used within a month

Lemon is good for our skin because it has the capability to lighten the skin complexion. It contains vitamin C which can keep skin healthy and fresh.

Tomato & Sea Salt

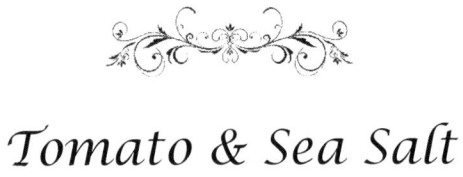

Ingredients
- 1 tomato
- 1 tablespoon sugar or sea salt
- ½ teaspoon almond oil
- 2-3 drops of essential oil (any)

Method
1. Chop tomatoes into rough, but very small cubes.
2. Add the sugar and mix well to make a paste.
3. Pour the almond oil, and 2-3 drops of any essential oil into it.
4. Mix well.

TO USE
- ON YOUR FACE: Apply to the face and massage in circular motions for 1 minute. Rinse well with water.
- ON YOUR HANDS: Massage into your hands and fingernails for 1 minute. Rinse well.

- ON YOUR LEGS AND FEET: Massage in circular motions for a few minutes. Rinse well.
- ON YOUR BODY: Massage in circular motions for a few minutes. Rinse well and moisturize.

*Use on the same day

Tomato has the capability of treating broken or uneven toned skin. it is also anti-aging for skin.

Vanilla, Coffee & Sugar

Ingredients

- ¼ cup finely ground dry coffee
- ½ cup sugar
- 2 tablespoons virgin coconut oil
- 2 tablespoons almond Oil
- ½ teaspoon natural vanilla extract

Method

1. Place the coffee and sugar in a bowl.
2. Add the oils and vanilla extract.
3. Mix well to make a thick paste.
4. Store in an air-tight container and keep it in fridge.

TO USE

- ON YOUR HANDS: Massage into your hands and fingernails for 1 minute. Rinse well with warm water.
- ON YOUR LEGS AND FEET: Massage in circular motions for a few minutes. Rinse well.

- ON YOUR BODY: Massage in circular motions for a few minutes. Rinse well and moisturize.

*Scrub needs to be used within a month

Coffee is proves to be life extender for skin. it is also a protector from dangerous UV rays.

Lemongrass & Olive Oil

Ingredients
- 2 tablespoons sea salt
- 1 tablespoon olive oil
- 4-5 drops of lemongrass essential oil

Method
1. Combine salt and olive oil to form a thick paste.
2. Add the lemongrass oil and mix well.

TO USE
- ON YOUR HANDS: Massage into your hands and fingernails for 30 seconds. Rinse well.
- ON YOUR LEGS AND FEET: Massage in circular motions for a few minutes. Rinse well.
- ON YOUR BODY: Massage in circular motions for a few minutes. Rinse well and moisturize.

*Use on the same day

Lemongrass is beneficial for skin because it is capable of killing bacteria and infections. It contains vitamins C as well which keeps the skin fresh and glowing.

Banana, Oats & Honey

Ingredients

- ½ a ripe banana
- 2 tablespoons oats
- 1 teaspoon honey
- 1 teaspoon milk

Method

1. Mash the banana in a bowl.
2. Add oats and combine well.
3. Add the honey and milk to make a mixture.
4. Mix all ingredients.

TO USE

- ON YOUR FACE: Apply to the face and massage in circular motions for 1 minute. Rinse well with water.
- ON YOUR HANDS: Massage into your hands and fingernails for 1 minute. Rinse well.
- ON YOUR LEGS AND FEET: Massage in circular motions for a few minutes. Rinse well.

- ON YOUR BODY: Let it rest on the body for 2 minutes before scrubbing. Massage in circular motions. Rinse well.

*Use on the same day

Banana is rich in vitamin C which acts as life for skin. Moreover, banana brings a unique glow to our skin.

Banana & Brown Sugar

Ingredients

- 2 bananas
- ¾ cup brown sugar
- 1 tablespoon olive oil

Method

1. Mash bananas in a clean bowl.
2. Combine with olive oil and sugar.
3. Mix well.
4. Store in an air-tight container and keep it in fridge.

TO USE

- ON YOUR HANDS: Massage into your hands and fingernails for 1 minute. Rinse well.
- ON YOUR LEGS AND FEET: Massage in circular motions for a few minutes. Rinse well.
- ON YOUR BODY: Massage in circular motions for a few minutes. Rinse well and moisturize.

*Use the scrub within 2 days

Optional: 1/2 teaspoon of vitamin E will help preserve the banana for longer. Than scrub needs to be used within a month.

Pomegranate & Sugar

Ingredients

- 1 pomegranate
- 1 tablespoon sugar
- 1/2 teaspoon grape seed oil

Method

1. Cut the pomegranate in half and deseed it.
2. Grind the seeds and mix with sugar.
3. Add the grape seed oil. Combine the mixture well.

TO USE

- ON YOUR FACE: Apply to the face and massage softly in circular motions for 2 minutes. Rinse well.
- ON YOUR HANDS: Massage into your hands and fingernails for 1 minute. Rinse well with warm water.
- ON YOUR BODY: Massage in circular motions for a few minutes. Rinse well and moisturize.

*Use on the same day

Watermelon & Mint

Ingredients

- ½ cup watermelon
- A few leaves of fresh mint or ½ teaspoon of dry mint
- 2 teaspoons of any oil
- 1 cup of coffee grounds

Method

1. Mix the watermelon and mint using a blender.
2. Add the oil and coffee grounds.
3. Store in an air-tight container and keep it in fridge.

TO USE

- ON YOUR HANDS: Massage into your hands and fingernails for 1 minute. Rinse well with warm water.
- ON YOUR LEGS AND FEET: Massage in circular motions for a few minutes. Rinse well.
- ON YOUR BODY: Massage in circular motions for a few minutes. Rinse well and moisturize.

*Use the scrub within 2 days

Optional: 1 teaspoon of vitamin E will help preserve the watermelon for longer. Than scrub needs to be used within a month.

Watermelon keeps the skin hydrated and toned.

Banana & Yogurt

Ingredients
- 1 banana
- 1 teaspoon yogurt
- 1 tablespoon honey
- 2 tablespoon almond powder

Method
1. Mash the banana in a bowl.
2. Add the honey.
3. Combine with the yogurt and almond powder.

TO USE
- ON YOUR FACE: Apply to the face and massage (with soft hands) in circular motions for 30 seconds. Rinse well with water.
- ON YOUR HANDS: Massage into your hands and fingernails for 1 minute. Rinse well.

- ON YOUR LEGS AND FEET: Massage (with soft hands) in circular motions for a few minutes. Rinse well with warm water.
- ON YOUR BODY: Massage (with soft hands) in circular motions for a few minutes. Rinse well and moisturize.

*Use on the same day

Yogurt keeps skin glowing and fresh. Moreover yogurt makes skin more elastic and removes dead cells from skin and treat broken lines if any.

Blueberry & Green Tea

Ingredients

- 1/3 cup fresh blueberries
- 1 teaspoon superfine sugar
- 2 tablespoons honey
- ½ teaspoon green tea

Method

1. Mash blueberries with the fork.
2. Blend blueberries with the honey, sugar and green tea.

TO USE

- ON YOUR FACE: Apply to the skin, covering the face and neck area. Leave the mixture for 15 minutes. Massage in circular motions for 30 seconds. Rinse well with water.
- ON YOUR HANDS: Massage into your hands and fingernails softly for 2 minutes. Rinse well

*Use on the same day

Sugar, Lemon & Olive Oil

Ingredients

- 1 lemon
- 2 tablespoons sugar
- 1 tablespoon olive oil

Method

1. Finely grind the sugar and put in an open bowl.
2. Cut the lemon in a half, removing the seeds.
3. Dip the lemon halves in the ground sugar.
4. Add the olive oil and mix well.

TO USE

- ON YOUR LEGS AND FEET: Massage in circular motions for a few minutes. Rinse well.
- ON YOUR BODY: Massage in circular motions for 2 minutes. Rinse well.

*Use on the same day

Orange & Oatmeal

Ingredients

- 3 tablespoons finely grated orange peel
- 2 tablespoons sea salt
- 3-4 drops of orange essential oil
- 3 tablespoons oatmeal
- 2 tablespoon ground flax-seed
- Olive oil

Method

1. Mix all the above ingredients together, except the olive oil.
2. Store in an air-tight container.
3. Using just a little at a time, mix the mixture with some olive oil to make a thick paste.

TO USE

- ON YOUR LEGS AND FEET: Massage in circular motions for a few minutes. Rinse well with warm water.

- ON YOUR BODY: Massage in circular motions for a few minutes. Rinse well.

*Use on the same day

Egg Shell & Cream

Ingredients

- 3 egg shells
- 1 teaspoon cream

Method

1. Toast the egg shells in a pan for 20-25 seconds so that it turns crisp and all the moisture evaporates.
2. Grind the shell into powder and mix with fresh cream to make a paste.

TO USE

- ON YOUR FACE: Apply to the face and massage in circular motions for 2 minutes. Rinse well with water.
- ON YOUR HANDS: Massage into your hands and fingernails for 2 minutes. Rinse well.

*Use on the same day

Sea Salt & Olive Oil

Ingredients
- 2 tablespoons sea salt
- 2-3 drops of tea tree essential oil
- 1 tablespoon olive oil

Method
1. In a bowl, take 2 teaspoons of sea salt.
2. Add the tea tree oil for antibacterial properties.
3. Mix well with enough olive oil to make a mixture of sufficient density.

TO USE
- ON YOUR BODY: Massage in circular motions for a few minutes. Rinse well and moisturize.

*Use on the same day

Olive oil keeps skin firm, toned, soft and smooth. It is a best moisturizers for your skin.

Coffee & Honey

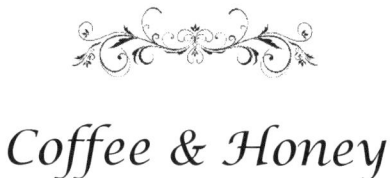

Ingredients

- 2 teaspoons grounded coffee
- 2 teaspoons honey
- 1 tablespoon coconut oil

Method

1. Mix well the grounded coffee and honey in a bowl.
2. Add the oil. Stir well.

TO USE

- ON YOUR FACE: Apply to the skin, covering the face and neck area. Massage in circular motions for 1 minute. Rinse well with warm water.
- ON YOUR HANDS: Massage into your hands and fingernails for 1 minute. Rinse well.
- ON YOUR LEGS AND FEET: Massage in circular motions for a few minutes. Rinse well.

*Use on the same day

Coconut & Brown Sugar

Ingredients
- 1 tablespoon melted coconut oil
- 2 tablespoons brown sugar

Method
1. Mix brown sugar in the coconut oil to make a thick mixture. (The ratio can be changed to acquire a thicker density).

TO USE
- ON YOUR HANDS: Massage into your hands and fingernails for 1 minute. Rinse well with warm water.
- ON YOUR BODY: Massage in circular motions for a few minutes. Rinse well.

*Use on the same day

Coconuts increases blood circulation and prevents skin cancer.

Oats, Honey & Grapefruit

Ingredients

- 4 tablespoons oats
- 2 tablespoons honey
- 2 tablespoons olive oil
- 4-5 drops of grapefruit essential oil

Method

1. Crush the oats to smaller grains.
2. Add the honey, olive oil and grapefruit oil.
3. Stir all ingredients well.

TO USE

- ON YOUR LEGS AND FEET: Massage in circular motions for a few minutes. Rinse well with warm water.
- ON YOUR BODY: Let it rest on the body for 2 minutes before scrubbing. Massage in circular motions. Rinse well.

*Use on the same day

Oats are best to remove dryness from skin. They are good for treatment of acne too.

Lemon, Sugar & Honey

Ingredients

- 1 lemon
- 1 tablespoon olive oil
- 1 tablespoon honey
- 3 tablespoons brown sugar

Method

1. Mix brown sugar, honey and olive oil in a bowl.
2. Add the juice from a fresh lemon.
3. Mix well.

TO USE

- ON YOUR LEGS AND FEET: Massage in circular motions for a few minutes. Rinse well with warm water.
- ON YOUR BODY: Massage in circular motions for a few minutes. Rinse well.

*Use on the same day

Kiwi & Sugar

Ingredients
- 1 kiwi
- 2 tablespoons sugar
- 1 tablespoon olive oil

Method
1. Blend the kiwi a little that the seeds are still existing.
2. Add remaining ingredients and mix well.

TO USE
- **ON YOUR FACE:** Apply to the skin, covering the face and neck area. Massage in circular motions for 2 minutes. Rinse well with warm water.
- **ON YOUR HANDS:** Massage into your hands and fingernails for 1 minute. Rinse well.
- **ON YOUR LEGS AND FEET:** Massage in circular motions for a few minutes. Rinse well.

*Use on the same day

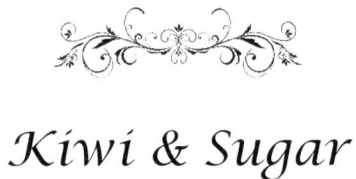

Strawberry, Honey & Almond

Ingredients

- 6 large strawberries
- ½ cup honey
- 1 cup sea salt
- 1 cup brown sugar
- 1 tablespoon almond oil
- 1 teaspoon vitamin E (it will help preserve the strawberries)

Method

1. Mix the salt and sugar together.
2. Mix the honey with the oil and vitamin E and pour into the salt & sugar mixture.
3. Mix thoroughly.
4. Blend strawberries for a while and add to the scrub.
5. Store in an air-tight container and keep it in fridge.
6. You can use some as a lip scrub.

TO USE

- ON YOUR FACE: Apply to the face and massage in circular motions for 1 minute. Rinse well with water.
- ON YOUR HANDS: Massage into your hands and fingernails for 1 minute. Rinse well with warm water.
- ON YOUR LEGS AND FEET: Massage in circular motions for a few minutes. Rinse well.
- ON YOUR BODY: Massage in circular motions for a few minutes. Rinse well.

*Scrub needs to be used within a month

CONCLUSION

Scrubs made up of natural ingredients unlike commercially produced scrubs acts positively on human skin and give no harm to it. Moreover, in order to have a healthy, young and glowing skin, homemade scrub is a must. Use your own scrubs, save money and stay beautiful.

I hope this book was able to increase your knowledge about why human skin needs to be scrubbed, how often and how. Moreover, this book contains 30 effective homemade scrubs recipes so that you don't have to apply commercially produced scrubs. Make your own scrubs using natural ingredients and keep your skin away from chemicals of commercially produced scrubs. Stay young by using homemade body and facial scrubs.

If you find this book extremely of help, sharing it with your friends and loved ones will be greatly valued.

Thank you and good luck!

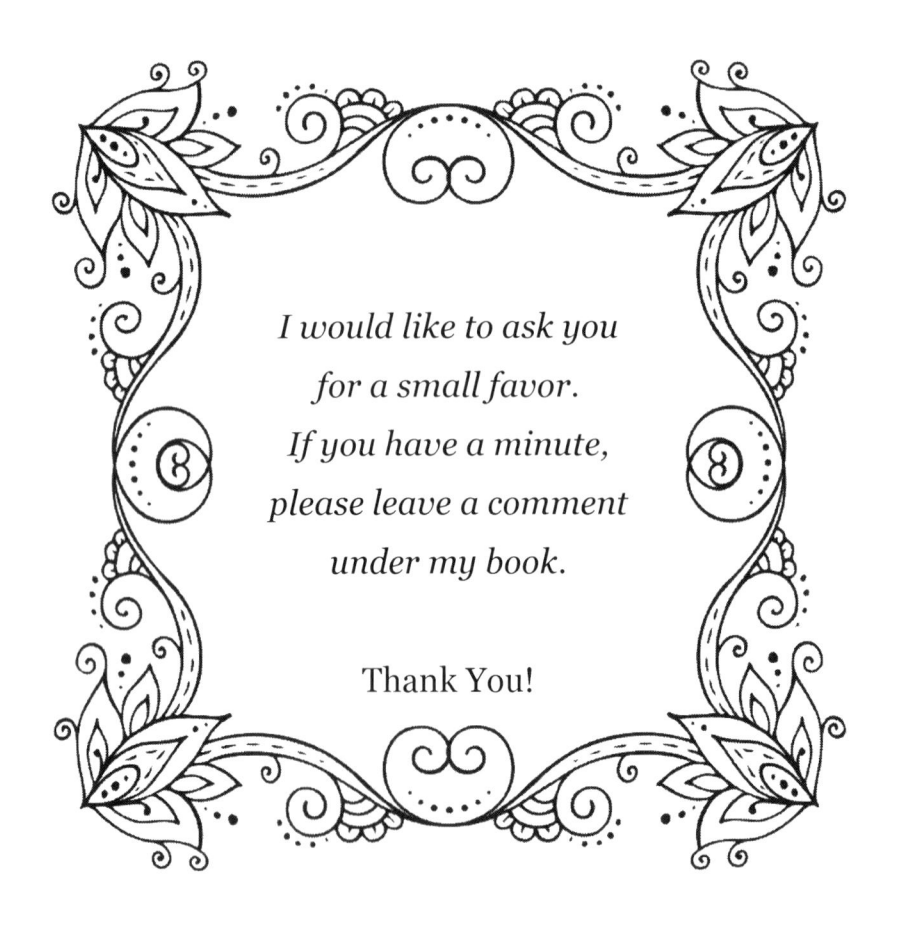

I would like to ask you for a small favor. If you have a minute, please leave a comment under my book.

Thank You!

CHECK OUT MY OTHER BOOKS

Bellow you will find my other books that are popular on Kindle.

Health & beauty:

Bath Bombs: Fizzy World Of Bath Bombs, Amazing Recipes To Create Beautiful And Creative Bath Bombs

Natural Hair Care Guide: How To Stop Hair Loss And Accelerate Hair Growth In A Natural Way, Get Strong, Healthy And Shiny Hair Without Chemicals

Essential Oils Guide: The Ultimate Guide To Essential Oils For Weight Loss, Stress Relief, Aromatherapy, Beauty Care, Easy Recipes For Health & Beauty

Essential Oils For Pets: Essential Oils For Dogs: 40 Safe & Effective Therapies And Remedies To Keep Your Dog Healthy From Puppy To Adult

Essential Oils For Cats: Safe & Effective Therapies And Remedies To Keep Your Cat Healthy And Happy

Anti-Aging Skin Care Secrets: Younger Skin Without Scalpel And Botox. Discover How To Rejuvenate Your Skin Quickly And Maintain A Youthful Appearance

Orchids care:
Orchids: Growing Orchids Made Easy And Pleasant. The Most Common Errors In The Cultivation Of Orchids. Let Your Orchids Grow For Many Years

[Phalaenopsis Orchids Care: 30 Most Important Things To Remember When Growing Phalaenopsis Orchids, How To Give The Best Life To Your Plants](#)

[Orchids Care For Hobbyists: The Advanced Guide For Orchid Enthusiasts](#)

[Orchids Care Bundle (Orchids + Orchids Care For Hobbyists): Growing Orchids Made Easy And Pleasant + The Advanced Guide For Orchid Enthusiasts](#)

[Phalaenopsis Orchids Box Set 2 in 1: Phalaenopsis Orchids Care + Orchids Care For Hobbyists](#)

[Orchids Care Bundle 3 in 1: Orchids + Orchids Care For Hobbyists + Phalaenopsis Orchids Care](#)

Speed Reading Guide For Beginners:
[Speed Reading Guide For Beginners: Get Your Fast Reading Skill The Easy Way. Simple Techniques To Increase Your Reading Speed In Less 24 Hours](#)

You can simply search for the titles on the Amazon website to find them.

Best regards!

Printed in Germany
by Amazon Distribution
GmbH, Leipzig